GW01048599

Pelvic Floor Physical Therapy Series:

Book 3

Your Pelvic Health Book

A Guide to Pelvic Floor Awareness, Bladder Health, Bowel Health, Sexual Health, and Changes throughout Your Lifetime for People with a Vagina and/or Uterus

By Jen Torborg, PT, DPT

MEDICAL DISCLAIMER

None of the content in this book constitutes medical advice, nor is it a substitute for personalized health care. It is intended for informational and educational purposes only and is not to be construed as medical advice or instruction. If you have concerns about any medical condition, diagnosis, or treatment, you should consult with a licensed health care provider. If you are experiencing a medical emergency, you should call 911 immediately.

Jen Torborg assumes no responsibility or liability for any consequences resulting directly or indirectly from any action or inaction you take based on the information in or material linked to this book.

ARTWORK

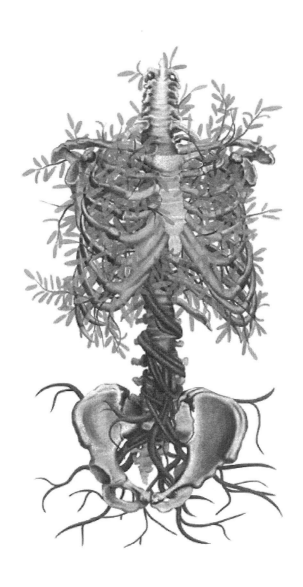

Cover design artwork by Ana-Maria Cosma

CONTENTS

INTRODUCTION

Normalizing bodily functions lessens shame and increases confidence.
—Melissa Pintor Carnagey, LBSW, founder of Sex Positive Families

The above quote sums up one of the main reasons why I'm writing this book. There are so many things I didn't know about my own bodily functions until I studied to become a physical therapist, and even more things I didn't know about "down there" until I specialized in becoming a pelvic floor physical therapist. One of the biggest lessons I've learned from my own experience and that of my clients' success has been that knowledge is power. With more awareness of our bodies, we can hopefully prevent many problems from occurring or at the very least understand when to reach out and ask for help.

This book isn't going to cover every single topic about your anatomy and physiology or what is normal versus concerning, but it will be a start in the right direction. Hopefully, I can provide you with some insight from a physical therapist (PT) point of view as to what's up down there. Our bodies change as we age, as we go through hormonal changes, as we change physically and mentally, and as we encounter trauma and surgeries. The more we can have awareness about this area of our body, our pelvic region, the better quality of life you may lead.

Many of the topics in this book were not talked about in my family while growing up. I didn't hear teachers or coaches talk much about this. I don't remember any of my health care providers giving me much education on what's normal and what to expect when it comes to pee, poop, sex, and life changes. Even as a high school athlete and a physical therapist, there was still not a lot of discussion about how the pelvic floor muscles play a role in our physical well-being and performance or how bowel, bladder, and sexual dysfunctions may play a role in our overall health. I think this lack of discussion comes from combination of lack of knowledge in the general public and health care professionals as well as a lack of comfort or willingness to discuss the subject.

But we can change this. Let's talk about our pelvic floor. Let's talk about bladder and bowel health. Let's talk about what a positive sexual health experience can be. Let's discuss the changes that can happen throughout a lifetime. The more we know, the more we can feel secure in our bodies. Let's share this information with our friends, our kids, our parents, and our community.

I'm Jen Torborg, a physical therapist specializing in pelvic health with a passion for sharing what I know with others. Just so you are aware I am a white, cisgender female who lives in rural northern Wisconsin. I am a very active, able-bodied person who loves to be outdoors and often uses nature as therapy. I aim to take what is common knowledge in the pelvic health community and make it more accessible to the general public. My first two books were directed towards pregnancy and postpartum health.* My aim with this book is to broaden the discussion of pelvic health to a wider range of ages and will include changes throughout the life cycle including menstruation and menopause. This book is for people with a vagina and/or uterus. I recognize that not all people will have both body parts, so not all parts of this book may be relevant to you.

Because of the limitations of my own professional experience thus far, this book does not cover information specific to children under the age of five or information specific to individuals with disabilities. However, there are many pelvic physical therapists and other health and wellness professionals that specialize in working with these populations, and it would be beneficial to consult with one who does for an individual approach due to the wide range in abilities and unique circumstances.

I will do my best throughout this book to remove cisnormative terminology while talking about pelvic health since anatomy and gender are completely different.

I use an asterisk sign* throughout this book to denote that the resource I'm providing or quoting uses cisnormative language in their content.

Enjoy!

XO
Jen

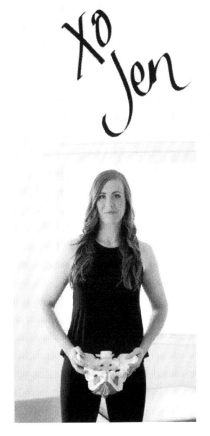

Photo credit: Kelsey Lindsey

CHAPTER 1:

ANATOMY AND PHYSIOLOGY 101 OF YOUR PELVIS: KNOWING WHAT'S UP DOWN THERE

Let's start with an anatomy lesson so that we can have an idea of what I'm referring to when I mention certain organs, muscles, bones, and other anatomy. The more we know about what our body parts are called in scientific terms, we can better describe accurately to health care professionals and others who might need info about what's going on down below. I will be going over anatomy related to vulvas, vaginas, and uteruses. Many people with vaginas are women, but some are men or nonbinary. Some vaginas are created surgically, and some people refer to their body parts with different words than those I mention.

Approximately 1.7 percent of the population is born as a variation of intersex, meaning they may have a combination of internal or external genitals, sex chromosome composition different from XY or XX, and/or variations in hormone levels.

- Intersex Society of North America answers FAQ and provides resources and support for those dealing with intersex conditions (link in Resources Appendix).

Whether you are intersex or not, know that when you see pictures in an anatomy textbook, it might not always look exactly like yours. Many times, these pictures are used to easily identify various anatomy features, but in real life there are all sorts of variations. For examples of the wide variety of vulvas, check out the *Great Wall of Vagina* artwork* or the *Labia Project* blog* (links in Resources Appendix). However, if you ever have a sudden, unexplained change in the appearance of your anatomy, that may be a reason to bring it up with a health care provider to rule out anything problematic.

I recommend learning the scientific terms for pelvic anatomy so that you feel informed about what many health care providers and educators are referring to. If you do prefer different terms for your body, that is okay and that is your choice completely. You may still find it helpful to compare with the anatomy terms, so if you need to explain any issues to a professional or talk through something with a partner, you have some common ground to translate your terms.

> Some people's bodies will not match any available diagrams, and it's important to know that it does not mean there's something wrong with their bodies, but that the system is narrow and flawed and *should* include them. (Jasper Moon, CPM, LMT)

The following diagrams and pictures do not show all variations of possible anatomy, nor do we dive into important anatomy such as your nervous system, vascular system, lymph system, or all the organs involved in your abdominal and pelvic region. This was done for simplicity of bringing awareness to this area, but keeping things brief and relevant. We will go through basic bladder, bowel, sexual/ reproductive, and pelvic floor muscle anatomy and physiology. This section will give you a basic intro to the anatomy and physiology of some pelvic parts with further descriptions given in later chapters.

A great idea for getting in tune with your own body is to draw your own diagrams or color in drawings of the pelvic anatomy variations. See my attempts at drawing the sexual/reproductive anatomy included later in this chapter. Have fun with it. Included in the Resources Appendix is a link to a coloring book by Heather Edwards, PT, founder of Vino and Vulvas™ called *Important Parts: A Coloring Book for the Crotch Enthusiast.*

General anatomy of the pelvic region in someone with a vagina and uterus

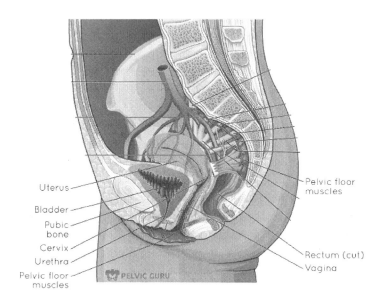

Uterus
Bladder
Pubic bone
Cervix
Urethra
Pelvic floor muscles

Pelvic floor muscles
Rectum (cut)
Vagina

Permission to use copyright image from Pelvic Guru, LLC.

14

The image above is included to help orient you in the pelvic region as to where the bladder, rectum, vagina, uterus, and pelvic floor muscles are in relation to each other. The following sections will go into more depth of each system.

BLADDER ANATOMY AND PHYSIOLOGY

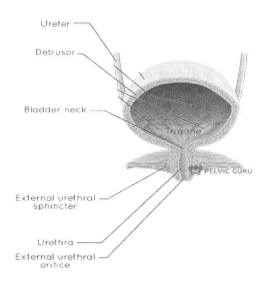

Permission to use copyright image from Pelvic Guru, LLC.

The urinary bladder sits just behind and above the pubic bone. Urine is first made in the kidneys and then travels to the bladder via the ureters. The bladder's job is to store urine until you're ready to go. When you are ready to urinate, your bladder muscle (detrusor) squeezes, the sphincters open, and out comes the urine through your urethra.

BOWEL ANATOMY AND PHYSIOLOGY

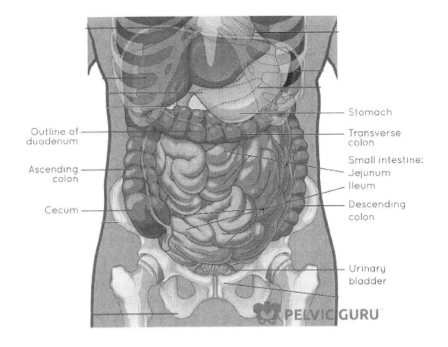

Permission to use copyright image from Pelvic Guru, LLC

Each section of bowel is made up of muscles and valves that help push food through in a process called peristalsis. The food travels from the stomach to the small intestine (duodenum, jejunum, and ileum) then makes its way through the large intestine (ascending, transverse, and descending colon). During this process the gut is absorbing some fluids and nutrients as well as processing and discarding waste. After the bowels have processed the nutrients, the remaining waste (stool/feces/poop) makes its way into the rectum. The brain receives a message once the waste arrives here that it's time to empty. The pelvic floor muscles and anal sphincters keep the poop and gas in until you're ready to release.

SEXUAL/REPRODUCTIVE ANATOMY AND PHYSIOLOGY

Next, we are going to go over what is typically referred to as your sex or reproductive anatomy, but remember that sexual experiences can include a lot more than these parts of your body. More on this in the sexual health chapter.

The parts of a vulva (external anatomy) include the labia (lips), clitoris, opening of the urethra, opening of the vagina, and anus.

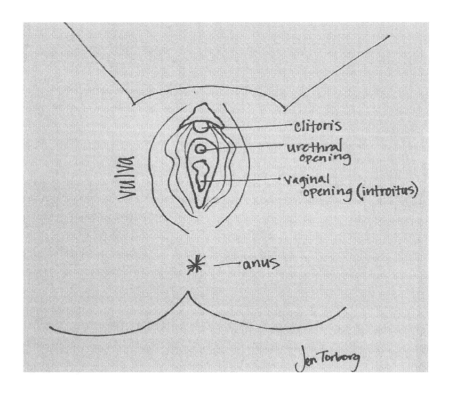

The internal anatomy includes the vagina, cervix, uterus, fallopian tubes, and ovaries. More on the physiology of this region in the menstruation section.

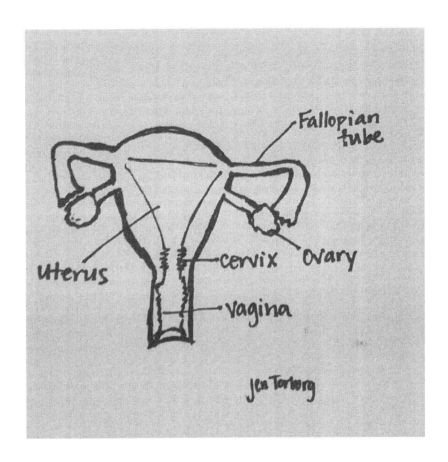

PELVIC FLOOR ANATOMY AND PHYSIOLOGY

The superficial pelvic floor muscles consist of the bulbospongiousus, ischiocavernosus, and superficial transverse perineal muscles.

The deeper pelvic floor muscles include the levator ani (iliococcygeus and pubococcygeus) and puborectalis muscles.

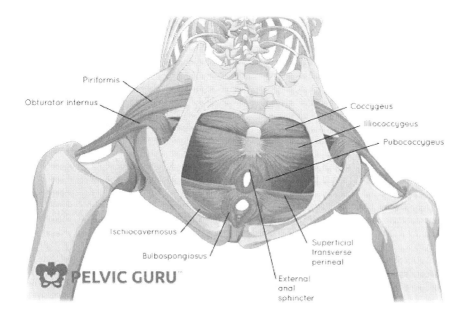

Permission to use copyright image from Pelvic Guru, LLC

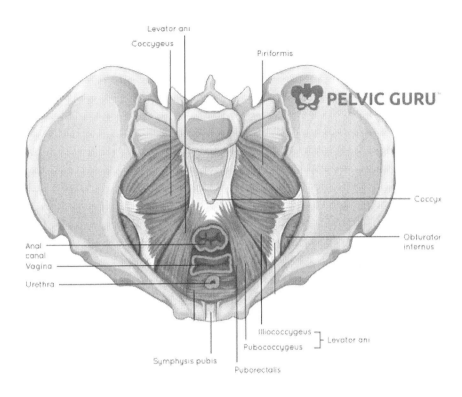

Levator ani
Coccygeus
Piriformis

PELVIC GURU

Coccyx

Obturator internus

Anal canal
Vagina
Urethra

Illiococcygeus
Pubococcygeus
Levator ani

Symphysis pubis
Puborectalis

Permission to use copyright image from Pelvic Guru, LLC

PHYSIOLOGY: PELVIC FLOOR, BREATH, POSTURE

As we move on to the pelvic floor, my aim is to explain how you can have better awareness of your breathing, pelvic floor muscles, and posture and relate that to your pelvic health. Many fitness professionals, coaches, and PTs are willing to talk about your core muscles and engaging your abs, but not many include your pelvic floor or breathing. Even at a young age, it is a disservice to you to not talk about your pelvic floor muscles pertaining to your awareness of this region and its effect on the performance of your body.

Your pelvic floor's function includes supporting the previous pelvic organs discussed—bowels, bladder, sex organs—and keeping these parts up and in your body. The pelvic floor plays an important role in keeping urine, gas, and poop inside of you until you're ready to go. It also plays a role in your sexual function.

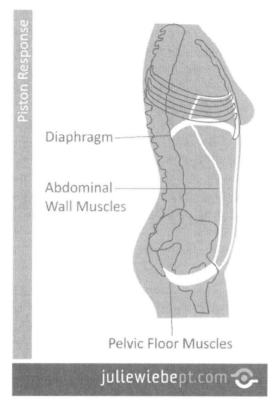

Illustration courtesy of Julie Wiebe. Used with permission.

Your core from my perspective refers to the innermost layer of muscles like the core of an apple or the core of the earth. In this sense, your core is made up of your pelvic floor muscles as the bottom foundation, your diaphragm (breathing muscle) as the roof or top (and this truly extends all the way up to your glottis [in your throat]), your transversus abdominus muscle (deep abdominals), and your multifidi (back muscles).

The concept of a pressure relationship between the diaphragm and the pelvic floor (and much more!) is taught as Piston Science created and owned by Julie Wiebe, PT. For over 20 years, she has been integrating these concepts and strategies into movement, function, and all forms of fitness including running, CrossFit, and more. Julie has also been an advocate for empowering people to pursue fitness in the midst of pelvic health and pain issues. She is internationally recognized for pioneering the integrative approach that is now widely relied upon by physical therapists and fitness professionals including me. Her information is used with permission. For more information about Julie, please visit her website, blogs, videos, and online courses. Links are located in the Resources Appendix.*

DIAPHRAGM BREATHING

Your diaphragm is the breathing muscle along the bottom of the ribs and the muscle that represents the roof of the core. Let's check in with your ability to take a nice, full, symmetrical breath—not just a chest or belly breath.

Take a breath in, and you can feel your ribs expand in all directions—to the front, to the sides, and to the back. A cue for this can be visualizing tree rings expanding, an umbrella opening, or the outward rippling of water when you drop a stone into it.

When you exhale and let the air out of your body (mouth or nose), let your ribs sink back down.

- *Inhale = gently feel ribs expand in all directions.*
- *Exhale = feel ribs sink back down.*

One way to add your breath to movement is to exhale on the exertion as to decrease the total pressure inside your body. You do not always need to do this, but if you encounter something particularly heavy or exerting or if you're working on trying to improve your pelvic floor control, this may be a helpful starting place. As you move your body from a sitting position to standing, while you lift a heavy object, while you bend down to pick something up, or while you reach for something, practice exhaling by blowing the air out of your mouth during the exertion. Take a full breath in to prepare followed by an exhale and move at the same time. This is an easy way to optimize the pressure inside your body and start getting your breathing, pelvic floor, and lower abdomen to coordinate again. Some cues that might help you remember to do this without making it a forceful exhalation and to avoid gripping your abdominals would be to pretend you are cooling soup on a spoon or blowing out through a straw when you move.

POSTURE

Changing up your posture throughout the day, being able to maintain a posture as needed, and moving in all different ways is great for your overall health. As I explain some ways you may improve upon your posture, remember that variability in posture is more important than trying to always hold an ideal posture.

Try to find a relatively neutral pelvic position some of the time. You don't want to tuck your tailbone/butt under and have a flat back all the time, but you also don't want to untuck to the extreme and arch your back to the max all the time. Go between those two directions a few times, and then try to find the middle ground. Doing this motion of tilting your pelvis back and forth or in circles a few times a day can be a useful movement for your pelvic health, especially if you sit a lot.

Now that your pelvis can move more easily, try to align your ribs over your pelvis. This will optimize your body's pressure system inside the core (diaphragm on top, pelvic floor on the bottom). Ribs over pelvis means not leaning so far back that your ribs are flared forward and not so rounded forward in your chest and shoulders that there's no room in the core. Again, find a middle ground and move your body as needed.

PELVIC FLOOR

Your pelvic floor muscles are those that connect from the pubic bone in the front to the tailbone in the back and your sit bones side to side. They are muscles that wrap around all three openings—urethra, vagina, and anus—and attach to various depths inside your pelvis. It is a group of muscles that work together to keep your organs up and inside of you, to keep you from leaking, and to provide support and stability.

To begin connecting with your pelvic floor, find the diaphragm breath we just talked about and a comfortable posture. Add a relaxation of the pelvic floor with your inhale and a contraction of the pelvic floor with your exhale.

Here are some visualizations that work for some people and may work for you.

To focus on relaxing, visualize your pelvic floor:

- letting go
- melting like butter
- opening like a flower

To focus on contracting your pelvic floor, visualize yourself:

- stopping from peeing
- stopping from passing gas
- pulling the pubic bone and tailbone up and into your body
- pulling the sit bones up and into your body

- pretending to close your vaginal opening around a kidney bean and lifting the bean up and into your body

As you're doing a pelvic floor contraction, try your best not to use your butt cheeks, squeeze your thighs together, hold your breath, squeeze your upper abs, or strain and bear down.

Start these pelvic floor exercises in isolation in all different positions: lying down, sitting, standing, on your hands and knees. Try them while in the shower, before going to bed, or whenever is convenient for you to pay attention to the quality and really focus on what's happening.

Combine these various cues for contraction and relaxation of the pelvic floor muscles with your breathing practice:

- *Inhale = relax pelvic floor muscles*
- *Exhale = contract pelvic floor muscles*

As you connect with this area and start to feel stronger, start to add the concept to movements: getting up from the chair, lifting objects, and bending down to pick something up from the floor. Add this concept to your exercise routine: squats, lunges, push-ups, pull-ups, etc. The strategy of *inhale + relax* with rest or the easy part of a movement, then *exhale + contract* on the hard part of a movement or exertion can be applied to all sorts of rep-based movements. Add this concept to a few repetitions with the focus on quality.

When it comes to physical activities that aren't rep-based such as walking, running, biking, or swimming, you want to be able to feel yourself find a full breath and that your pelvic floor can follow your breath and contract and relax as you need it to. Rather than timing out exactly where to breathe and squeeze, your focus becomes simply connecting with your breath and pelvic floor during these activities and noticing that you're not tensing or contracting the whole time, but that you also have the ability to contract as needed for support too.

Over time, you will want the ability to contract, relax, and lengthen your pelvic floor in all types of positions and movements. Lengthening your pelvic floor is used while having a bowel movement, but remember to breathe. Don't strain or push.

You'll want to be able to contract not only on an exhale but also with an inhale. You'll want to vary the length of your contractions so that you can work all of your different muscle fiber types. You'll want to be able to do quick contractions (one to two seconds) of your pelvic floor muscles, not associating them with breathing. Don't hyperventilate! And you'll want to perform endurance contractions (more than 10 seconds) while you continue to breathe in and out. Don't hold your breath.

You also want to vary the intensity you're contracting at. We don't want to squeeze our maximum amount all the time. Do we do that constantly with other muscles or only go for max reps in the gym? No. We often seek variety. So, the majority of the time, you're probably only going to contract at 50 percent effort or less. Check in with your ability to squeeze and lift at all different amounts.

To maintain quality strength of your pelvic floor, you will want to avoid constant clenching of your abdominals and pelvic floor. It's so important that this area, like all other muscles, can find a balance between activation and relaxation. If you aren't sure if you are performing pelvic floor exercises correctly, seek out feedback from a professional such as a pelvic floor physical therapist.

The goal of performing pelvic floor exercises and having an awareness of this area is really like all muscle groups. For the most part, your body is magical and amazing and knows just what to do. However, for some people because of previous cueing, habits, body changes, and so on, we need to bring a purposeful awareness to this part of our body. If you are experiencing any pain, leakage, pelvic heaviness, or other pelvic floor, abdominal, back, or hip symptoms, you may need to get specific about how your pelvic floor and all body parts related to this area are functioning. Check in with your body to see how well you're able to contract, relax, and lengthen your pelvic floor muscles. How's your breathing? How's your posture? How's your ability to vary your posture and move in many different directions and positions? If you have concerns about any of these symptoms or feel limited in your movements and daily functions, consider seeking out a physical therapist specializing in the pelvic floor or other fitness or movement professionals with experience in this area of your body. The Pelvic Guru global directory of pelvic health professionals and other physical therapist locators can be found in the Resources Appendix.

GENERAL HYGIENE AND CHOICES FOR DOWN BELOW

I decided to add a few basic tips on hygiene and choices about down below in this section. It is healthy to wipe from front to back after voiding or having a bowel movement so that you don't bring any anal bacteria towards the vagina or urethra. Try not to let moisture get trapped in this area for long. Clean with water and pat dry if you're sweaty, experiencing leakage, or having other moisture issues. Wear breathable clothes or underwear when possible. When cleaning your vulva, just use warm water. No scrubbing or douching is necessary. Be careful about soaps, wipes, and other products. You may want to avoid products with toxic chemicals and fragrances. Fragrances and certain chemicals can irritate your urethra, vagina, and anus.

Choose to have your body hair however you want. If you want to let things go wild and natural, if you want to trim, if you want to shave, if you want to wax or laser, it's your own choice, and although there are a few health pros and cons for the various decisions of what you do with your hair, it is totally up to you.

RECAP

1. Learn about the anatomy and physiology of the bladder, bowel, and uterine systems.
2. Know what your pelvic floor is and how to contract, relax, and lengthen your pelvic floor muscles.

3. Understand how your breathing and posture can affect your pelvic floor.
4. Know a bit about how hygiene and product choices can affect your pelvic health.

CHAPTER 2:

BLADDER HEALTH

Hopefully, you now understand a bit about what your bladder anatomy looks like and the basic concept of how urine goes from your kidneys to your bladder and then leaves your body. This chapter is going to bring in more details about what is the normal, healthy state of the bladder and what could be problematic as it pertains to your bladder health.

Most of the time I see clients for bladder problems, it's because we were never taught what are healthy voiding habits. So here are some generalizations about the healthy state of a bladder. And although everyone has their own variations of normal, these are some suggestions about what habits to follow as they pertain to maintaining healthy bladder function.

Most bladders can hold about 2 cups of fluid before it needs to empty (16 oz., 400–500mL). Most people feel an urge to go when your bladder is about 40 percent full, although many other things can affect feeling an urge earlier or later than that. Keeping in mind you want to drink about 6 to 8 cups of water steadily throughout your day, you will probably be going to the bathroom every two to four hours to urinate during your waking hours. At night, depending on how many hours you sleep, most people won't have to wake up at all to void, and some maybe need to do that just once per night. This can definitely change during pregnancy due to total blood volume and baby pressing on bladder. And it may increase slightly as we age to once to twice per night after age 65.

When you urinate, take your time and relax. Don't push, strain, or rush yourself. You hopefully will have a nice constant stream of urine. You want to have an easy time starting the flow, and you want to feel like your bladder is empty at the end of voiding. Normal urination is not supposed to hurt. If you're sitting to urinate, it is best to sit on the toilet seat. Don't hover above it. Hovering above the seat creates tension in your pelvic floor muscles and makes it more difficult for you to fully relax and release all of your urine. Sit down on public toilets. Use toilet paper or a seat cover if that makes you more comfortable, but don't avoid urinating or hover because you think there are germs on the toilet seat. The likelihood of you catching anything from a toilet seat is slim to none.

So now that you have a general sense of what are healthy habits. What can be problematic? If you encounter any of the common but not normal issues listed below, consider seeking out an individualized assessment and treatment approach for your unique situation with a trained pelvic floor physical therapist. There are also many medications that have side effects that can contribute to bladder dysfunctions (frequency, urgency, and leakage). Speak with your pharmacist or primary provider if you have concerns about your medications effect on your bladder.

URINARY FREQUENCY AND URGENCY

If you have to urinate sooner than every two hours on a regular basis, this could be considered urinary frequency and could become a problem if it starts to interfere with your daily activities and quality of life. If you hold longer than four hours on a regular basis, ignore urges to go because you're busy, restrict fluid intake because your job, school, or other circumstances don't allow you to go when you need to, this could become a problem that leads to UTIs (urinary tract infections), urgency, or leakage. You don't want to go "just in case" on a regular basis. Going sooner than two hours, holding past four hours, or going "just in case" may sometimes happen and is not anything to worry about, but if you repeat these habits regularly or feel you don't have the ability to control or change them, this could be problematic. Sometimes you may not have access to restrooms or know when your next chance to void might be. But in most cases, with awareness of your habits and a little planning, you'll be able to decrease your "just in case" voids and improve the timing between your voids. When you feel an urge to pee or feel like you're just going out of habit rather than a true filling urge, ask yourself: When did I last go the bathroom? (Was it just 15 minutes ago, or has it been more than two hours?) How much did I drink and what did I drink? When will I get a chance to go again?

For most people, just water as your fluid intake is best for your body and bladder. Use your tap water if possible and avoid use of plastic water bottles. Plastic water bottles can be expensive and are destructive to the environment. Plastic is a potential hormone disruptor to your body. Unfortunately, not everyone has access to clean water, especially free clean water. Consider testing your tap water at home for safety and see if there is a filter system you can buy that makes it safe enough to drink so that you don't have to pay for bottled water. I realize this is a privileged thing to suggest because of cost, but consider the money you would be spending on bottled water and other beverages and see if there's a way to make some of the water from your home safe. If not, do you have somewhere in your community you can refill jugs of clean water for free? Consider getting a water bottle you can take with you so that you are able to drink clean water frequently throughout the day.

There are various recommendations pertaining to water intake. Here are the top three:

- Drink 6–8 cups of water per day (8 oz. = 1 cup)
- Drink half your body weight in ounces of water per day. Example: you weigh 160 pounds ÷ 2 = drink 80 oz. of water daily.
- Drink water when you're thirsty.

Things that may affect your water intake are activity level, how much you sweat, and climate.

Considering our bodies are made up of about 70 percent water, it's pretty important stuff. Water helps with many body functions including breathing, eyesight, digestion, regulate body temperature, bladder and bowel function, protection of organs and tissues, brain function, physical recovery, and more.

Many other fluids (and certain foods) have the potential to irritate your bladder lining, causing you urges to go more frequently. This doesn't mean fluids other than water are necessarily bad or unhealthy, it just may mean it's worth paying attention to, especially if you're struggling with urgency, frequency, or dehydration. An easy first step is drinking some water around the times you drink other fluids. The added water can help dilute the irritant and keep you hydrated, especially while consuming diuretics such as coffee and alcohol. Soda, tea, milk, juice, and anything with sugar or artificial flavorings or sweeteners may contribute to bladder irritation. These might be fluids you wish to consider decreasing or avoiding if you are having any bladder issues.

If you're struggling with suppressing urinary urges, think back to when this first became a problem and think about when in your day it is the worst. Are there any patterns you can recall? If the problem came on over time (in other words, you used to be able to suppress your urges without difficulty, or it only happened occasionally), chances are you and your circumstances created this habit, but you can intentionally work to reverse it.

The first goal is to decrease your sense of urgency. You will want to decrease your desire to sprint to the bathroom. When you feel a strong urge, you may want to rush to the toilet, give in right away, and have difficulty getting your mind off the thought, but oftentimes this just makes things worse.

If you have a strong urge to urinate, try

1. Stopping right where you are. Don't move, walk, or squirm.

2. Distract your mind: count backwards from 100 by sevens, go through your to-do list or grocery list, name all the trees or birds you can think of.
3. Take gentle breaths in and out.
4. Do some gentle pelvic floor contractions.
5. Wiggle your toes.

With any luck, your urge will probably stop or at least decrease in intensity within a few seconds to minutes. The mind is powerful. Once the urge has dissipated, you can ask yourself: When's the last time I went to the bathroom? How much have I drunk since then? And if it feels appropriate to urinate, go ahead and make your way *calmly* to the bathroom. If it feels like you're experiencing an urge out of habit or triggers but not that your bladder is actually full, try waiting a little longer to go.

Find a balance with your bladder habits in listening to what your body is telling you and what you now understand to be healthy habits. Your habits will change based on what you're eating and drinking, what your schedule is like, access to bathrooms, etc., but hopefully, this gives you a general idea of what to expect when it comes to voiding.

If you feel you are not fully emptying your bladder and you're already taking your time in the bathroom, consider the "double void." This would be rocking your pelvis forward and backward while sitting on the toilet, standing up and then sitting back down again, or standing up walking around just a few steps and then sitting back down again. Sometimes this allows remaining urine to shift and come forward if it didn't have an easy exit (prolapse, tight muscles, etc.).

URINARY LEAKAGE

Urinary leakage can happen at any age—young and old and anywhere in between. Urinary leakage, also known as urinary incontinence, is the involuntary loss of urine. There are a few different types of urinary leakage: urge, stress or exertional, mixed, functional, and nighttime. Urinary leakage can happen in a teenage athlete, in someone pregnant or postpartum, in someone with a busy or demanding job, in someone going through menopause, or recently post-surgery. *Urinary leakage is common but never normal.* But there's help. Pelvic floor physical therapy can be very helpful in treating leakage and can be one of your first choices in treatment. While working through stopping urine leakage, make sure you are using protection created specifically for urine rather than menstruation (pads, diapers, or underwear such as the ICON brand).

Urge urinary incontinence occurs when you have a strong urge to urinate and then leak before you're able to make it to the bathroom. One of the main ways to first address this type of leakage is to address why the urge is happening and work to suppress and retrain habits surrounding that urge. Treatment may consist of taking a good look at your voiding frequency, hydration habits, bladder irritants, causes of urge, as well as assessing what's going on with your pelvic floor muscles and addressing any muscle imbalances—too weak, too tight, or difficult coordination with breathing or movements.

Stress urinary incontinence, now often called exertional incontinence, has more to do with increased pressure on the bladder and pelvic floor internally. The pelvic floor muscles are usually not strong enough, are holding too much tension, or not coordinated well enough to respond appropriately. This type of leakage can happen with coughing, sneezing, laughing, lifting, exercising, jumping, moving from sit to stand, or other forms of exertion and pressure changes in the body. Treatment of this type of leakage may involve having a pelvic physical therapist assess your breathing patterns, posture, pelvic floor muscle activation, relaxation and timing with movement and exertion. When treating urinary leakage, there is usually much more to it than strengthening your pelvic floor muscles. And sometimes strengthening might not be the right choice at all. You may need to work more on relaxation or coordination. It's helpful to perform your pelvic floor exercises with the actual movements or causes of your leakage, not just sitting or lying down in isolation repeating rep after rep without real-life scenarios to challenge yourself.

Mixed incontinence is a combination of urge and stress/exertional, so both treatment approaches discussed would be part of your plan to better health.

Functional incontinence is when someone has a hard time getting to the bathroom because of physical and/or mental concerns. This could be difficulty moving to the bathroom, balancing, undressing, etc. Treating functional incontinence may involve improving your pelvic floor control and urge suppression patterns as well as addressing how to improve your ability to get to the toilet and undress safely and efficiently. The practice of timing your voids may be helpful with this type of leakage.

Nighttime leakage can occur for many reasons and can sometimes be harder to treat because you're sleeping and therefore have decreased conscious awareness to think through the previously discussed treatment ideas. Usually, if daytime habits and control issues are improved, they can help with nighttime patterns. Also, being able to decrease the volume of the bladder fullness at night can help.

If you wake up frequently during the night to void and/or are leaking during this time, consider

1. Decreasing or stopping fluids two to three hours before bed
2. Elevating your feet to heart level or higher for 15 minutes around two hours before bed
3. Pumping your ankles up and down during the evening before bed

These tips can help decrease the total fluid in your system before bed and improve the blood circulation of your legs before lying down in bed, so there's a chance you will go one more time before bed or go a larger volume before going to sleep.

There are many reasons why some people will experience bladder problems during their lives. Some can be changed and prevented with knowledge and awareness and others may be due to genetics, medical complications, surgeries or injuries, or past history. Even the way you were toilet trained by your parents or caregivers and allowed to go or not go during school or jobs can have an effect on your bladder habits later in life. If there was any punishment or rewards associated with your bladder habits, that may also have an effect on your awareness and bodily autonomy. Sexual abuse may have an effect on your urinary functions. If you are struggling with bladder dysfunction, there is hope and there is help.

RECAP

1. Consider creating habits where you urinate on average every two to four hours during the day while aiming to drink about 6 to 8 cups of water spread out throughout your day.

2. Urinary frequency (going sooner than every two hours) is common but not normal and can be treated.

3. Holding your urine for more than four hours on a regular basis or restricting water intake can be problematic for your bladder health.

4. Urinary urgency can be balanced between listening to your body and using your education about what's healthy to decide if it's appropriate to go. Sometimes you may choose to delay the urge and other times calmly head to the bathroom.

5. Urinary leakage is common, but it is never normal, and there are multiple ways to treat it. Consider seeking out a pelvic floor physical therapist for an individualized approach.

CHAPTER 3:

BOWEL HEALTH

Bowel health is something I absolutely did not feel comfortable talking about as a kid. I was embarrassed to go in public restrooms, I ignored urges at school, and I most likely had some food sensitivities and stress contributing to my bowel habits, but I honestly didn't know anything could be done about them. My family and the majority of my friends didn't talk about poop. No one reiterated to me that everyone poops and it's a normal, healthy habit that happens on a regular basis. No one told me pooping shouldn't hurt. No one told me having a good quality bowel movement daily can be an enjoyable experience.

Until I went in to pelvic physical therapy, improved my nutrition, and bought a Squatty Potty®, I thought I was doomed to unpredictable poops that varied between diarrhea and straining, painful constipation. Thank goodness that wasn't the end of the story for me. Hopefully for you and your loved ones, this chapter will help clear up any confusion you have on pooping.

The Bristol Stool Chart helps to classify the consistency of poop on using seven descriptions. Types 1–2 are descriptive of constipation. Types 3–4 are ideal. Type 4 is the easy-to-pass long banana poop that you're aiming for. Types 5–7 explain the consistencies of diarrhea.

BRISTOL STOOL SCALE

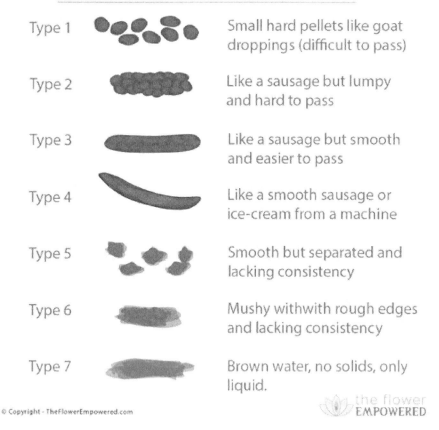

Type 1 — Small hard pellets like goat droppings (difficult to pass)

Type 2 — Like a sausage but lumpy and hard to pass

Type 3 — Like a sausage but smooth and easier to pass

Type 4 — Like a smooth sausage or ice-cream from a machine

Type 5 — Smooth but separated and lacking consistency

Type 6 — Mushy withwith rough edges and lacking consistency

Type 7 — Brown water, no solids, only liquid.

the flower
EMPOWERED

Illustration courtesy of The Flower Empowered. Used with permission.

It is ideal to have a bowel movement at least once per day. However, variations of normal could be anywhere from three times per week to three times per day. The important part is that you're staying pretty regular with your own bowel movement (BM) schedule and aren't experiencing any sudden, unexplained variations to less frequent or more frequent. Usually, BMs are healthiest when they fall within types 3-4 on the Bristol Stool Chart (pictured above) and feel easy to pass. Most people have a regular time frame that they feel they are ready to have a bowel movement when they pay attention to their emptying reflex such as after drinking a warm beverage in the mornings or 30 minutes after eating. When you feel the urge to have a BM, listen to what your body is telling you and head to the bathroom calmly when you get a chance. Your body will hopefully be able to keep the stool inside of you while you make your way to the bathroom. Upon sitting on the toilet, your BM will likely begin within a minute or so if everything is on track. Relax on the toilet and don't rush yourself. Your BM has the possibility to be easy to pass without straining or pain.

Ignoring the urge over and over because you're busy, don't have a bathroom near you, are uncomfortable going in the bathroom that is convenient to you, or are uncomfortable going with people around you could all contribute to bowel dysfunctions such as constipation.

A bowel movement doesn't have to take long to pass. It can be easy, pain-free, and feel good. You hopefully won't need to push or strain. If you do feel like you need to exert a little effort to lengthen the pelvic floor and get things out, try exhaling by blowing out air through your mouth. Do your best to avoid breath holding while on the toilet.

If you've ever experienced a BM on a really low toilet or squatting out in the woods, you may already know its typically much easier to pass a BM while you're in a squatting posture. This is the natural way our body was designed to poop. The squatting position helps relax our puborectalis muscle (one of the pelvic floor muscles) and allows a better angle for our stool to exit our bodies. If your toilet options include a standard height or raised height, you may want to consider a stool under your feet to mimic a squat position from the comfort of your toilet. Squatty Potty® is a brand of stools made specifically for this purpose, but any step stool, yoga blocks, books, or boxes can help get the job done. The goal is to get your knees higher than your hips, comfortably lean forward keeping your back straight so you don't tuck your tailbone, breathe, and poop. Just like with urinating, don't hover over a toilet to poop. Hovering will make it even harder to pass stool as you're tensing the pelvic floor muscles and doing the opposite of a relaxing squat. If you're concerned about the cleanliness of a bathroom toilet, put down some toilet paper or a seat cover.

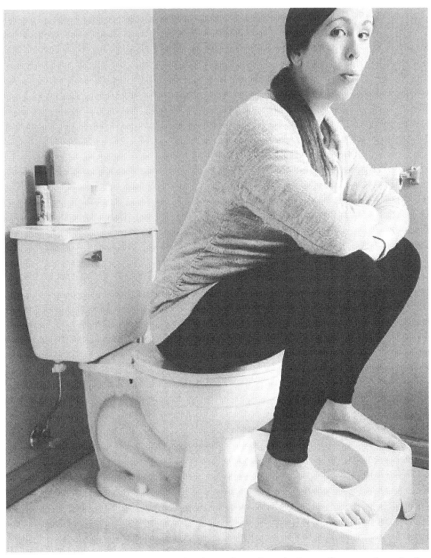

Use a Squatty Potty® (knees higher than hips), lean forward, exhale.

If you have aversions or embarrassments about pooping, consider where this feeling comes from and perhaps journal on this, talk to a therapist, or work with a pelvic floor physical therapist. Try to accept that everyone poops. It's a normal, healthy function. If you have concerns about the smell of your poop, consider purchasing a toilet spray such as Poo-Pourri to carry with you or have in your bathroom at home. You usually spray this before you have a BM, and it can help cover the smell of your poop. If sound is of concern for you, consider seeking out or asking if the bathrooms you typically use could play music to cover up the sound.

BOWEL CONCERNS

If you're spending long periods of time in the bathroom, straining or pushing to go, have irregular BMs, have hemorrhoids, pain with BMs, constipation, or diarrhea, you probably have some form of bowel dysfunction. Consider how some of the following underlying factors might be contributing to your bowel function:

1. Fiber and fluid balance
2. Possible medication involvement
3. Laxative abuse, long-term use, reliance, or tolerance
4. Food sensitivities, gut health
5. Sedentary lifestyle
6. Pelvic floor muscle ability to relax and coordinate
7. Scar tissue adhesions
8. Stress management
9. Lifestyle changes: traveling, pregnancy and postpartum, after surgery

A pelvic floor physical therapist can help you address many of the above-listed considerations. Consider talking directly to your primary provider and pharmacist about any medication and side effect concerns you have.

You may want to see someone with a specialization in nutrition for more detailed information, testing, and treatment programs to find out if you have any food sensitivities. The nutrition specialist may use an elimination diet of some sort or FODMAP diet temporarily while figuring out what's going on.

> FODMAPs are a group of [short-chain] carbohydrates (sugars and fibers) that are commonly malabsorbed in the small intestine. FODMAPs are abundant in the diet and can be found in everyday foods such as wheat, barley, rye, apples, pears, mango, onion, garlic, honey, kidney beans, cashew nuts, agave syrup, sugar-free gum, mints and some medicines, to name a few. Up to 75 percent of those who suffer with irritable bowel syndrome (IBS) will benefit from dietary restriction of FODMAPs. Research has shown the low FODMAP diet improves gastrointestinal (GI) symptoms (gas, bloating, pain, change in bowel habits) related to IBS. FODMAPs is an acronym that stands for fermentable oligosaccharides (fructans and GOS), disaccharides (lactose, milk sugar), monosaccharides (excess fructose), and polyols (sugar alcohols). What is the low-FODMAP diet? The low- FODMAP diet is a two- to six-week elimination diet that involves removing high FODMAP foods from the diet to assess whether FODMAP-rich foods are triggering your GI symptoms. The low FODMAP diet is a *learning diet* rather than one that you stay on forever. The goal of the diet is to help you determine your personal dietary triggers. After the low-FODMAP elimination diet phase, a dietitian will guide you on how to

reintroduce FODMAPs in a methodical manner to assess your tolerance to various FODMAP-containing foods. Many people will find they can liberalize their FODMAP diet restrictions and only need to restrict some high-FODMAP foods. The low-FODMAP diet should be implemented with the help of a FODMAP-knowledgeable dietitian to help you navigate the many nuances of the diet and to help you develop a personalized, well-balanced eating plan. Do not self-diagnose. If you are troubled by GI symptoms, be sure to consult with your doctor. (Kate Scarlata, RDN)

Good quality sources of fiber and the right amount of clean water can really make a difference in your stool consistency. The right combo of fiber can help bulk up your stool or help make it smoother to pass. Sources of fiber come from plants. These include fruits, vegetables, beans and legumes, grains, and nuts and seeds. General recommendations for fiber intake are around 25–35 grams, but you may have to make adjustments based on how the consistency of your stool is turning out. You need to find the right balance of fiber for you. It can help loosen stool and bulk up stool depending on how much and what kinds of fiber you're digesting. Hydration recommendations as mentioned in the urinary section are usually 6–8 cups (48–64 oz.) of water daily. Other recommendations can include 50 percent of your body weight in ounces of water or drinking when you're thirsty. You will probably need to increase your water intake if you're sweating a lot, in a dry climate, or are increasing your activity level. You may also want to look for ways to add gut healing foods to your diet such as probiotics, magnesium, and more.

Sedentary lifestyle can contribute to disruptions in a healthy bowel movement pattern. Walking, moving your body in ways that feel good to you, and changing up your posture and positions throughout the day if possible are great ideas to counteract this. Doing some deep breathing exercises can help massage your colon from the inside. Stretching the muscles around your pelvis, hips, abdomen, and back are all great ideas too. Some examples of stretches can include lying on your back and bringing one or both knees to your chest, child's pose yoga stretch, a supported deep squat, and many more.

If you're having trouble relaxing your pelvic floor muscles, this could contribute to pain with BMs and other bowel dysfunctions. This could be from tight muscles, areas of tenderness or pain, a neurological response to pain or fear, scar tissue, or decreased mobility in your joints. You can work with a pelvic floor physical therapist to release tension and improve mobility of your pelvic floor muscles and other structures around this region. The pelvic floor physical therapist may help you figure out what manual therapy and stretching is needed. There are definitely ways you can take charge of your body and follow through at home with what is taught to you.

Scar tissue adhesions from previous abdominal or pelvic surgeries or injuries could have an effect on how well your stool passes through your body. Working with a pelvic physical therapist or massage therapist specializing in this area may be helpful to decrease tension in this region, calm the nervous system, and improve blood flow and overall body movement.

Bowel massage can also be a great way to stimulate your body to get things moving. The goal is to apply pain-free pressure to the abdomen and sides of the trunk following your large intestine in the direction you want the stool to leave your body (through the rectum) on the left lower side of your body. You can make circle or stroking motions in this *clockwise direction,* or you can break it down into steps sometimes referred to as the ILU (I love you) colon massage. This just breaks up the massage into three parts but still follows a clockwise direction.

1. Top left to bottom left (I)
2. Then top right to top left to bottom left (L)
3. And then finally bottom right to top right to top left to bottom left (U)

Do five to 10 times in each direction once a day or as needed to get a BM going.

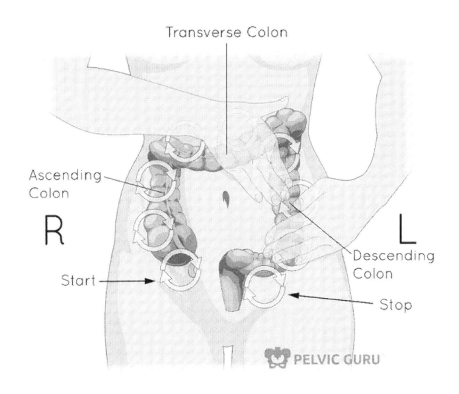

Transverse Colon

Ascending Colon

R

L

Descending Colon

Start

Stop

Permission to use copyright images from Pelvic Guru, LLC

If you're traveling or some of your daily habits are about to be disrupted, try to take control of whatever factors help you have your optimal bowel movements: hydration, quality nutrition and fiber intake, staying active, going for walks, and trying to time out your BM at the same time as your typical emptying reflex (mornings after a hot beverage or 30 minutes after a meal). Add in some diaphragm breathing and stretching. Consider a bowel massage if needed. And bring a Squatty Potty® or makeshift stool if you can. I often flip a bathroom garbage can and use that as my stool when I'm not at home.

The way we process or respond to stress can have a big effect on our physical bodies, especially the gut health and our bowel health. If you have difficulty finding ways to process and respond to stress in your life, consider journaling through it, write down ideas that bring you joy and help you work through stress, find ways to slow down and be present, breathe, meditate, and be mindful through decisions. Reach out to a therapist or other professionals in the healing arts to work through treatments and solutions to better respond to stressors in your life.

Let's talk a little more about gut health and its influence on your body.

> So, what causes [altered gut microbiota] imbalance in the first place? It's the overall stress load on the body over a period of time. For example, stress, individual genetic differences, and perceived threat which includes fear, hopelessness, and pain. Pain itself is both a sensory and emotional response to both a perceived and/or actual threat. Other things like diet, history of antibiotic use, constipation, and infections can also disrupt the gut microbiota. It's not uncommon to see a lack of gut bacteria diversity in individuals experiencing pelvic pain; especially low are the anti-inflammatory bacteria that help keep the peace. Here are four things you can do to help repair and restore your gut back to health:

1. [Consider trying] an anti-inflammatory diet (not a special diet fad; keep it simple). [...] Eat a variety of colorful, whole

foods per meal and double-check the ingredients (sugars can be sneaky). It's worth working with a functional medicine practitioner [and/or registered dietitian] to get an accurate picture of your gut health so you know which diet is right for you.

2. **Poop regularly.** Constipation and other bowel disturbances can disrupt the flora in your gut. Invest in a poop stoop or Squatty Potty® and drink plenty of water. General rule of thumb is to drink half your body weight in ounces.

3. **Chew your food slowly.** Your stomach doesn't have teeth. Chewing helps release digestive enzymes to break down and emulsify your food making it easier on digestion. So, for example, if you're eating something hard like an almond, you should chew it 20–40 times. Time to strengthen those muscles of mastication!

4. **Meditate.** Psychological stress stimulates the fight-or- flight response by releasing stress hormones into the bloodstream. Great in short doses, not so good for your health with prolonged stress. Over time these stress hormones can alter gut microbiota. Meditation helps regulate the stress response by stimulating the rest-and- digest nervous system, which reduces inflammation and helps maintain a healthy gut barrier function. (Dr. Susie Gronski, DPT, PRPC, WCS, WHC)*

Leaking gas or stool

Just like we talked about urine leakage in the previous chapter, gas and stool can leak out too. *This can be common but not normal.*

When referring to leaking gas, I'm talking about the involuntary loss of gas, not letting it go on purpose. If you're someone who always lets your gas go the moment it comes (because it certainly does feel better once its released), check to see if you have the ability to hold in the gas. Walk to another room (such as the bathroom) and then release. If you are able to control it and keep it in when needed, awesome. Then it's totally up to you whenever you want to let one go. If, however, you cannot stop yourself from holding back gas when you want to, then it may be important to work on your pelvic floor muscle strength and coordination using the information in chapter one and working with a pelvic floor physical therapist.

For fecal incontinence (leakage of stool), there are a few different things we would want to address more than just pelvic floor control. You would also want to take a better look at the consistency of your stool and see what can be done to help your rectum and sphincters sense when it's filling and what it's filling with (gas versus stool). You would also want to look at your bowel habits to see if we can optimize your patterns. It may be worthwhile, like most areas of the body, to not limit ourselves to just looking at the pelvic region but also a thorough screen of the spine, hips, and nervous system. And of course, check out your pelvic floor muscle control as well.

RECAP

1. Normal bowel movements occur regularly in frequency (usually at least once per day). They are soft and easy to pass, usually within a minute of sitting down on the toilet.

2. Bowel movements don't have to hurt, cause straining or pushing, take a long time to pass, or be too hard or too loose. If you are avoiding BMs or are fearful of having a bowel movement, reach out for help.

3. Improve your BMs by listening to your body, using a squat position on the toilet, staying active, drinking water, getting an adequate amount of fiber, and addressing stress management, food sensitivities, and any other concerns.

4. Leakage of gas and stool can be common but not normal. Seek out help with a pelvic floor physical therapist.

CHAPTER 4:

SEXUAL HEALTH

Sexual health encompasses much more than sex organs or penetrative intercourse, but we are going to focus mostly on the physical aspect of sexual health from the perspective of a pelvic floor physical therapist in this chapter. For further awareness around sexual health (perspectives from other fields), consider working with a sex education counselor or therapist. The folks at Planned Parenthood are also fabulous resources—the sex ed most of us never got in high school.

Sex in all its forms should be consensual. It should not be coerced. Sex can feel great. It doesn't have to be painful unless you are seeking to create that type of experience. Whether we're talking about solo sex or sex with partner(s), sex can be an enjoyable experience.

> Exploring one's own genitals is a valuable part of sexual health that often begins in childhood. Don't shame it! (Melissa Pintor Carnagey, LBSW, founder of Sex Positive Families)

Explore what feels like good touch to you. And don't forget that the brain is probably one of your most important pieces of your sexual experience. The more you understand about the anatomy of your own body and what feels good to you, the better your sex experience may be and the better you can communicate your needs to a partner. Did you know that most people aren't able to achieve orgasm through vaginal penetration alone, and that 70 percent or more need clitoral stimulation to orgasm? The clitoral complex is the center of pleasure for people who have it. People who can orgasm through vaginal penetration alone generally happen to have anatomy that allows the clitoral complex to be stimulated that way. Most of the rest of us need direct stimulation on the glans. Explore what feels good to you with touch of your hands and/or the use of toys.

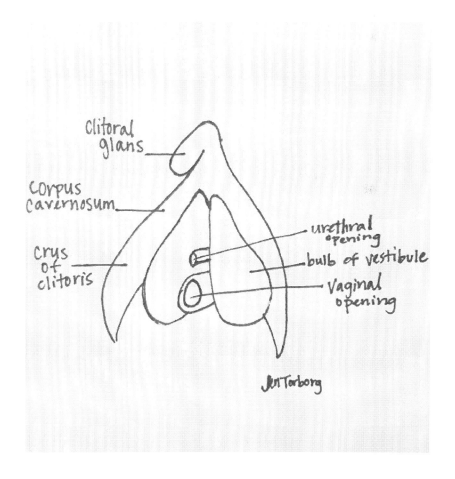

SELF EXPLORATION AND TOYS

There are many resources available for you to better understand this part of your body, what might turn you on, what feels good, etc.

Inclusive supportive sex guides include

- Health Line: LGBTQIA Safe Sex Guide
- Planned Parenthood: Sex and Relationships
- Human Rights Campaign Foundation: Safer Sex for Trans Bodies

There are many toys available that may help you have a satisfying sexual experience solo or with a partner if you are interested in it. Be aware of the materials of any toys you're using. Seek out high-quality materials and avoid toxicity in toys, which could cause irritation and contribute to pelvic pain. Consider choosing nonporous toys that are easy to clean (silicone, glass, metal). Glass and metal toys can be used with all types of lubricants. However, silicone toys cannot be used with silicone lubricant.

Epiphora explains on her blog post "Your Genitals Deserve Better: The Case against Toxic Sex Toys" (link in Resources Appendix), to look for body-safe toys. Watch out for PVC toys, porous toys that could harbor bacteria, paint that could chip off, and harmful additives. All anal toys should have properly flared bases. When looking for quality products she suggests to:

> Look for sex toys made of the same materials as kitchen tools: pure silicone, stainless steel, glass, sealed wood, aluminum, ceramic, stone, acrylic, and hard plastic. Buy from a trusted retailer.

Lubrication

Sometimes you need a little lubricant or a lot of it. There are moments in many people's lives where they may be on the drier

61

side or run out of moisture with friction or time. It's normal and expected to need time to become aroused enough to make your own lubrication, and even then it might not be enough to make things comfortable. Penetration before arousal can be painful or create microtears.

There are a lot of lubricant options out there, but my advice is to read the labels. Some lubricants that are well marketed can actually dry you out more or may have irritating additives and chemical fragrances causing a burning sensation. Look for options without glycerin or parabens, flavors, fragrances, or tingling effects. Opt for water-based or silicone-based lubricants (Slippery Stuff, Good Clean Love, Yes!, Sliquid Organics, Uber Lube), or consider coconut oil, olive oil, or vitamin E oil. Some oil-based lubricants break down latex condoms, and silicone lube destroys silicone toys, so make sure you know if everything you're using works well together. Generally, water-based lubricants work okay with most things.

When engaging in sex of any kind with other people, it's important to discuss HIV and STI status, protection, and testing. If you have a uterus and your partner makes sperm, also discuss the possibility of pregnancy. There are many hormonal and non-hormonal or barrier methods of contraception. Only condoms protect sufficiently against most STIs.

There is a wealth of resources located at the Sex Positive Families resources page including websites, videos, books, and tip sheets to strengthen sexual health and body awareness for all ages (link in Resources Appendix).

PAIN WITH SEX

First, we are going to talk about unwanted pelvic pain with sex, why it might happen, and what can be done to help improve it. The pain may be always present or only happen with touch. This painful touch could be external with toys, fingers, or oral stimulation. This touch could be internal with penetration by yourself, a toy, or a partner.

There are moments in life where sex may cause a slight discomfort: first time, adjusting to the new size of a partner or toy, returning to sex postpartum, fisting and size play, or returning to sex after a surgery. However, with good communication, any discomfort within pleasure will hopefully be brief (resolving within a few seconds or within a few sessions).

Some causes of pain during sex could be
- emotional or psychological causes: fear including anxiety about pregnancy, lack of education or knowledge, not being ready or comfortable or not wanting to be having this type of sex at all or right now or with this person, previous pain, previous trauma or abuse, etc.
- dryness or lack of lubrication
- pelvic floor tension
- changes in your pelvic region (after surgery, prolapse, etc.)

If sex is painful for some of the emotional or psychological reasons, your nervous system becomes heightened, and that can affect your pelvic floor muscles and other body systems. If you've experienced pain with sex before, have a history of trauma or abuse, or have any shame or guilt associated with sex, a specific sexual act, or your sexual attraction patterns, you may benefit from talking with a mental health therapist or sex counselor. You may benefit from increasing your knowledge by reading more about sex education, learning about how the body works, learning about contraception and protective options, and finding answers to other questions you may have to ease nerves.

From a physical perspective, you can work on improving your sexual experience with some of the advice I'm about to go through and with an experienced pelvic floor physical therapist or other professional specializing in this area.

GRADED EXPOSURE TO POSITIVE TOUCH

If your body perceives that something will be painful, regardless of whether there is actual tissue damage, it will most likely be painful. This section will cover advice on how you can get comfortable with your genitals yourself and if desired, with a partner. The progression you move through will be based on listening to your own body and what it's ready for.

Start with approaches to touch that you already know feel comfortable to you. Often, our lack of awareness, comfort, and confidence in knowing this part of our body may contribute to fear, pain, and tension we feel.

FEELING YOURSELF EXTERNALLY

Here's an exercise to consider if you feel ready:

Next time you're in the shower or have some time to lie down in a relaxed position, start by feeling your abdominal and pelvic region. Simply begin with the goal of feeling the tissues and muscles on the outside. If you have any scars in this region, bring some gentle touch and awareness to them. For some this may be easy. For others, it may be triggering. If you're not ready to touch your scars yet, skip this part for now. Feel around the rest of your abdomen, the sides of your torso, your low back, hips, butt, inner thighs. Feel the skin, the muscles, the bones. Get comfortable with your own hands touching your body. Add in some gentle stretching or yoga to target the muscles attaching around your pelvis (abdomen, back, hips, legs).

When you're ready, (this may be the same or a future session), move your touch to your genital region. Make sure to use a clean finger while doing so. Touch your external genitals, your vulva, clitoris, perineum, anus. If you are going to be exploring touch to both your vulva and your anus, it is okay to move from vulva to anus, but it is important to rewash your hands when moving from anus to vulva so that you don't bring anal bacteria to the vagina or urethra. Feel your way around externally and see if there are any painful areas. If so, work on gently touching that area in a way that does not cause pain. Use gentle touch in a slow, intentional way to increase your positive experience in self-exploration rather than pushing through pain.

FEELING YOURSELF INTERNALLY

When and if you feel ready to do so, progress by starting to feel internally. Do so gently with a clean finger. Begin by slowly inserting one finger into your vagina or anus. Use as much lubricant as needed. When you are entering the vagina or anus, it can be helpful to imagine the openings as a clock with 12:00 toward the urethra and 6:00 toward the tailbone. It is usually most comfortable to enter either opening at the 6:00 position. Hold there for a bit and simply sense how it feels. Slowly move your finger towards the right and the left. Take your time and try to see if this can be a positive or at least neutral experience. Do not push into pain. Take full breaths as you're doing this and think positive thoughts.

Advance to feel deeper and/or with more speed depending on your goals. Continue to feel in different directions and depths. Use different pressures. Feel your pelvic floor muscles internally: contract, relax, and lengthen. Feel your breath gently expand and contract these muscles at a low level naturally. Notice if there are any areas that feel tight or painful and slowly work to bring gentle touch and release to those areas.

Continue to bring positive touch internally and externally in any ways that you may want to encounter during sex. Use this time to be present with your body and your experience. Note if there are certain areas that you will want to be careful and mindful of while being with a partner. Only pursue this exercise as a positive, pain-free experience.

ADDING A PARTNER TO THE MIX

If you have a sexual partner(s) you'd like to include, consider the following exercise:

It can help to start this exercise with an open conversation at a neutral moment (not during a sexual encounter) about your pain, about going slowly, and speaking up if something doesn't feel right. You may not jump right back into positions, toys, or speeds you were used to previously. There may be different positions that are less painful and allow for you to feel more in control of the depth of penetration. Ohnut is a newer device on the market aimed to help control the depth of penetration for people experiencing deep pelvic pain. Rings are added to a penetrating partner's penis or toy. The same way you've worked through touching yourself slowly and intentionally may be something you want to work through with your partner. You may choose to start with only external stimulation. The more open and honest you can be, the more your partner may be able to help you into making this a positive, pain-free activity you'll continue to enjoy in the long run. Don't put pressure on yourself to orgasm right away. Find new ways to enjoy sexual touch rather than pushing through anything (friction, speed, positions, length of time) you're not ready for. You may want to follow up sex with gentle breathing, cuddling, stretching, ice, heat, or relaxing postures to calm your nervous system and relax your muscles.

ADDING THERAPEUTIC OBJECTS TO THE MIX

Other ways some people find helpful to advance through pelvic pain with sex is using external objects specifically created for the purpose of treatment and healing. You may want to work with a pelvic floor physical therapist or other bodywork providers specializing in this treatment to find the right size and choice for your goals.

- Dilators are designed for increasing the depth and/or circumference of your vagina or anus.
- A TheraWand is a tool designed to help you reach specific tender areas of muscles deeper in the pelvic floor via the vagina or anus.
- A vibrator (or other vibrating objects) can be used to help with healing tissue and scars externally and internally. It is also used to relax muscles and reduce pain.

There are lots of options to help you heal physically and emotionally. If one strategy, practitioner, tool, or technique doesn't work for you, you may find others are more helpful. As you work through the above steps, you will hopefully be able to return to sex pain-free.

You do not have to push through pain (if it is unwanted). There are specific ways a pelvic physical therapist, sex counselor, and other professionals can help you to work through the various reasons you may be experiencing pelvic pain. A pelvic physical therapist can help you better understand what's happening with your muscles, joints, and other tissues, and how the nervous system and brain is responding in a protective way and how to work through that.

OTHER IDEAS FOR PAIN RELIEF

Other helpful tips to work on calming down the nervous system and releasing tension in the pelvic floor and surrounding areas may include

- Breathing exercises
- Stretching: abdominal region, pelvis, lumbar spine, hips, legs
- Relaxation techniques: meditation, mindfulness, positive mantras, calming music
- Gentle yoga routines

RECAP

1. Sex should be consensual.
2. Sex can feel great and be enjoyable. Explore what feels good to you.
3. If sex hurts and it is not your desire for it to be painful, there could be a combination of things going on including physical and/or emotional causes.
4. Slowly introducing positive touch to your own body can help to build confidence about what feels good and what may need some time and work.

5. Work with a professional—mental health or sex therapist and pelvic floor physical therapist or another bodywork professional—to address components of pelvic pain.

CHAPTER 5:

CHANGES THROUGH THE LIFETIME

There are many unique changes our bodies will encounter throughout a lifetime based on our sexual anatomy, hormones, age, lifestyle factors, and more. This chapter is going to dive into some of these changes pertaining to people who have or had a uterus. This portion of the book will cover the basics of menstruation, pregnancy and postpartum, and menopause.

MENSTRUATION/PERIODS

I'll let Melissa Pintor Carnagey, LBSW, of Sex Positive Families give you the scoop of how and why periods happen:

> The basic rundown of the process is this: people with uteruses can bleed for a few days monthly. It is natural. It's not dirty or wrong. It can happen when an ovum (one of thousands of eggs that people with uteruses are born with) is not fertilized by a sperm. A sperm is the other half of what creates a human baby. Sperm is made in the bodies of people with testes. A sperm and an ovum can meet during some types of sex or with the help of a doctor. The blood that comes out of the vagina from the uterus is made up of natural parts like blood, cells, tissue and mucus. Those things were hanging out in the uterus as part of a lining that would have protected a fertilized ovum as it grew into a fetus or baby. If an ovum is not fertilized, the lining which

looks likes blood, leaves the uterus through the vagina. It can take around three to seven days for all of the lining to exit. It generally does this process monthly as long as an ovum is not fertilized. During menstruation a person can feel other things like cramping, bloating, or changes in mood because the body is working hard and doing amazing things. It's important that people who are menstruating are supported and respected.

We may want to educate our children—both those presumed to have a uterus and those presumed not to (it's probably best to start before age eight)—so they aren't caught off guard if they themselves (or peers) start bleeding and are confused or scared about what's going on.

Although there can be mild forms of discomfort during your period, normal periods aren't supposed to hurt. If you're experiencing pain during your period, you can try to decrease its intensity with some of the treatment techniques I'll discuss below.

If you are experiencing moderate to severe pain, especially pain that's interfering with your quality of life or ability to participate in school, jobs, taking care of yourself or your family, you can seek out help for further testing and treatments. While you're talking to your primary provider, ask for a referral to a pelvic floor physical therapist to learn about some individual treatment ideas to help decrease your pain. This is a great first line of treatment before introducing medications or surgical interventions. Birth control medications sometimes mask period pain symptoms instead of treating the cause.

Treatment ideas for period pain may include
1. Pain relief measures: heat, TENS unit, essential oils
2. Pelvic floor relaxation
3. Stretching
4. Posture tips
5. Breathing
6. Relaxation techniques such as meditation
7. Hydration
8. Quality nutrition and decreasing foods that could cause inflammation (and foods that you may be sensitive to)
9. Exercising in ways that feel good to you
10. Pelvic floor physical therapy, massage therapy, acupuncture, chiropractic, other healing arts

Keeping track of when you get your period, how long it lasts, any symptoms you feel, and if you feel any signs of when ovulation is occurring (discharge, cramping near ovaries, height of your cervix) may be helpful to better understand your body. This can help you understand when to expect your period and how to know if there are changes in your cycle. There are many free apps to track your period on your phone, or you could write it down on a calendar.

There are four phases of the menstrual cycle: menstruation, the follicular phase, ovulation, and the luteal phase.

Each phase of your monthly cycle brings about different physical and emotional feelings, kind of like the seasons in nature. There is a reason that nature has darker seasons of cold and quiet and seasons of growth and lots of light. Our bodies are very similar to the natural environment around us, constantly ebbing and flowing, and we [can] all learn to honor our own powerful internal cyclical nature. (Nicole Jardim, The Period Girl)*

PERIOD DYSFUNCTIONS SUCH AS ENDOMETRIOSIS, POLYCYSTIC OVARIAN SYNDROME, AND MORE

Endometriosis, Polycystic Ovarian Syndrome (PCOS), and other period dysfunctions will mostly likely require you to dive deeper into figuring out what's going on with professional help in addition to the suggested treatment ideas for general period pain. Nutrition can be a very important piece of the puzzle while working with period dysfunctions. For example, many people with endometriosis have bowel issues, which have the possibility of clearing up with a low inflammatory diet. The Period Repair Manual by Lara Briden, ND, is a good resource for people with endometriosis, PCOS, and other period dysfunctions.

Endometriosis is a disease where tissue similar to but not the same as the lining of the uterus is found elsewhere throughout the body. Symptoms can include but are not limited to painful menstrual cramps, IBS, bloating, back pain, hip pain, and painful sex. Unfortunately,

74

endometriosis also causes reactive pelvic floor muscle spasms and adaptations throughout your body and central nervous system that may require interventions beyond surgery for the disease. Even after excision surgery, the gold standard in endometriosis care, [people] may continue to experience symptoms and this is where a pelvic health specialist can become a very important member of the multidisciplinary team treating endometriosis. With the average diagnostic delay of seven years for [people] with endometriosis, too many have suffered far too long without relief. Some [people] have been told the pain is all in your head, or you wait for a doctor to fix you after so many treatment options fail. Perhaps you are afraid to try just one more thing because it has been such a difficult journey. Don't be afraid. The refreshing thing about pelvic health physical therapy is that you are the most important member of the treatment team. Success with physical therapy is a partnership between you and your therapist. Many [people] are surprised the relief they feel from treating musculoskeletal issues contributing to their pain. Learning how connected the body is and how endometriosis has affected everything from the nerves to the core muscles to their sex lives is tremendously empowering. Likewise, having techniques to use when at home during a pain flare and having another professional in your corner reminds you that despite all the things that have happened to your body, you have influence over your own daily life. You are not your pain, and you can get better! (Dr. Sallie Sarrel, PT, ATC, DPT)*

Dr. Sallie Sarrel is a pelvic physical therapist who was diagnosed with endometriosis after two decades of pelvic pain. Her website (link in Resources Appendix) contains many helpful links including links for more information and support groups for those suffering from endometriosis.

> PCOS stands for polycystic ovary syndrome. For reasons that are largely unknown, [people] with polycystic ovary syndrome often have at least one of several hormonal imbalances. Usually [people] with PCOS make levels of sex hormones like testosterone that are too high. [People] with PCOS often have insulin resistance. Insulin resistance is an early predictor of diabetes and is basically a milder form of diabetes. When you have insulin resistance, you have trouble transferring the sugar from your blood into your cells because the insulin (the hormone that transfers sugar from blood to cells) has a difficult time doing its job. If insulin resistance is left alone, eventually it will progress to become diabetes, putting people with PCOS at risk for serious complications like heart disease, blindness, and amputation. If you have any of the following symptoms, you might have PCOS: weight gain, acne, heavy or darker face, chest, or body hair, ovarian cysts (these can be very painful if they rupture), bladder pain, difficulty getting pregnant, or depression. . . . If you're beginning to see yourself in this picture, don't worry. The great news is that PCOS can be easy to improve with some simple nutrition and lifestyle shifts. Many [people] return to having completely normal

hormone levels using nutrition and lifestyle medicine approaches alone. PCOS is best taken care of with a great team approach focusing on nutrition and healthy lifestyle as a foundation. (Dr. Jessica Drummond, DCN, CNS, PT)*

Jessica Drummond's website is an awesome resource for using nutrition and a holistic approach in healing many pelvic pain and period dysfunctions. Her website info for the Integrative Women's Health Institute and their signature program, The Pelvic Pain Natural Relief Method™, are linked to in the Resources Appendix.

PERIOD PROTECTION CHOICES

You have a choice in what type of period protection you might choose to help contain the blood discharging from your body so you can go about your day. You would probably benefit from limiting chemical exposure to all parts of your body for health reasons, but especially your vulva and vagina. Period products made with chemicals such as bleach and other toxins may contribute to pelvic pain. Many commercial tampons and pads can fall under this category, so it's good to understand what the products are made of that you are choosing to put into your vagina or near your vulva.

Here are some considerations for *reusable* period options which help create money savings opportunities and decrease what you're putting into the landfill:

- Menstrual cups such as Diva Cup, Mooncup, Luna Cup, and many more. Link to a comparison chart and a quiz to find out which cup is right for you by "Put a Cup in It" is located in the Resources Appendix. Look for medical grade silicone cups and use the flame test to check quality if you are unsure.

- Reusable pads such as Party in My Pants, or make your own
- Reusable period underwear such as THINX®

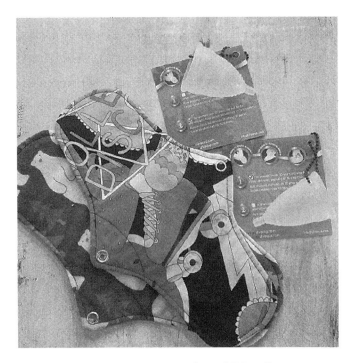

Party in my Pants pads and Diva Cups

If you prefer a disposable option, consider an *organic, bleach-free* tampon or pad for less chemical exposure such as

- Lola
- Cora Organics
- Seventh Generation

Normal periods aren't supposed to hurt, but because of the amount of work your body is doing and your hormonal fluctuations, you may want to slow down and be specific about what types of activities you engage in or how full you choose to fill your schedule the week of your period. Some of us may embrace their menses as a time of magic and connection, while others may just do their best to get through. Regardless of where you fall on this spectrum, if you need more individualized help or have questions, please do reach out to a pelvic floor physical therapist, a sex educator, functional nutritionist, or another health and wellness professional specializing in this area.

PREGNANCY AND POSTPARTUM

So we've already talked about the menstrual cycle and what happens when the egg is not fertilized. If an ovum released during ovulation does get fertilized by a sperm, it will generally make its way down the fallopian tube (usually three to four days) and enter the uterus. There it will attempt to attach to the lining of the uterus (implantation). If the implantation is successful, the uterus lining will thicken, and the cervix will be plugged with mucus. Inside the uterus at the site of implantation, the cells will continue to divide and multiply and eventually develop into a placenta and a baby. The hormone hCG, released by the embryo, tells the body to maintain its uterine lining rather than shed it, and begin preparing the body for growing a baby.

Bodies change during pregnancy as you are growing a baby inside you, and bodies change postpartum as you heal after birth (with both cesarean and vaginal births).

You have options when it comes to your health and choices in pregnancy including where you want to birth (home, birth center, hospital) and with whom present (doctor, midwife, doula, partner). If you're experiencing any aches or pains, urinary leakage, pelvic heaviness, or other changes during pregnancy, talk to your prenatal care provider and ask if help from a pelvic physical therapist would be appropriate. Although not all people will need it, everyone deserves the right to respectful prenatal and postnatal care, pelvic physical therapy, doula services, and lactation consulting during pregnancy and postpartum.

After childbirth, it can be really helpful and healing to rest when possible in the beginning (ideally at least two weeks of rest in/around the bed) as your body heals. Then slowly and intentionally over time, return to your daily activities, exercise, sex, and any other goals you have pain-free and without leakage or other discomforts. Again, if something doesn't feel right, don't shrug it off. Consider asking for help.

My first two books have detailed information for this time in a person's life from a pelvic floor physical therapist perspective. Keep in mind that my first two books do include cisnormative language that genders body parts. It was written with cisgender women in mind, and much of the information may be relevant to other folks who are pregnant or postpartum, but I recognize in retrospect that there are ways in which some people might not feel seen. I would highly recommend reaching out to Jasper Moon, CPM, LMT, who offers evidence-based, trauma-informed, queer and trans-competent reproductive care in the greater Portland, Oregon, area. There is a link to their website in the Resources Appendix.

Here's a quick recap of what these two books cover.

Book 1, Your Best Pregnancy Ever: 9 Healthy Habits to Empower You in Pregnancy, Birth, and Recovery

Whether this is your first pregnancy or your fifth, this pregnancy book aims to empower you with healthy habits from a pelvic floor physical therapy standpoint. Sure, there are already pregnancy books out there that are filled with every possible detail you may want to know, but not everyone has time for that. This book is different from the others. This pregnancy book is a quick, easy read for my pregnant people out there wanting to start developing some healthy habits right now. You'll find plenty of options and variations for you to make these habits your own. This book was written to give you insight into what people mean when they say, "just listen to your body." It's meant to give you a way to listen to that voice and know how to modify or ask for help. The tips provided in this book allow you to embrace this time and connect with your body in a healthy and inspiring way.

You can apply these easy-to-follow habits to have your best pregnancy, birth, and recovery:

1. **Breathing:** Learn about how embracing your breath can affect your body and mind including your breathing during

labor and birth. As your body changes, continue to utilize diaphragm breathing (with as much expansion that feels possible and comfortable) as a healthy habit for relaxation and pressure management. Exhale on exertion to decrease pressure inside your body.

2. **Pelvic floor exercises:** Understand how knowing more about your pelvic floor has the potential to improve your health. Research shows that working on pelvic floor exercises can improve your bladder control during pregnancy and postpartum. You will benefit from knowing how to contract, relax, and lengthen your pelvic floor muscles and how to add this to your everyday life while you're pregnant.

3. **Common versus normal:** Know the difference between what is common (happens frequently) versus what is normal (healthy state of the body). For example, a lot of people pee their pants during pregnancy and after childbirth, but leakage of urine is never normal. By understanding what is common versus normal during pregnancy and postpartum, you can reach out for help, attempt to prevent dysfunction, or modify activities as needed.

4. **Exercise:** Learn how to move in ways that feel good to you, modify as needed throughout pregnancy to avoid pain, leakage, and feelings of pelvic heaviness. Staying active in ways that feel good can improve your outcomes now and during your recovery.

5. **Sleep:** Sleep is important to your overall health, especially while you're growing a baby. Prioritize sleep and learn easy-

to-adopt strategies to improve your sleep if you're struggling with this.

6. **Nutrients:** Increase your knowledge about how to nourish your body and your baby with quality food. Drink plenty of water.

7. **Posture and alignment:** Understand how to adjust your posture to decrease pain in a variety of sustained positions and in movements for your best pregnancy experience. Overall, try to move your body in a variety of positions.

8. **Self-care:** Learn about why it's beneficial to make self-care an approach and a philosophy versus another item on your checklist.

9. **Preparing for birth and recovery:** While preparing for birth you may consider perineal massage and stretching starting around 35 weeks. You may want to be prepared with a variety of ideas for labor and birthing positions and ideas of how to breathe during birth. Also, start to get an idea of what to expect postpartum so that you can plan for rest and healing.

Book 2, Your Best Body after Baby: A Postpartum Guide to Exercise, Sex, and Pelvic Floor Recovery

This book was written for your postpartum healing. Like the first book, the goal is to give you insight into what "just listen to your body" really means. The book will help you learn how to modify or ask for help when returning to exercise, sex, and everyday activities. The suggestions provided in this book allow you to connect with your healing body so that you can return to activities in an intentional way.

Go slowly in the first few days and weeks postpartum as your organs, muscles, and tissues heal. I recommend the two weeks in/around the bed, two weeks around the house, two weeks around the community as a very generalized idea about how to gradually resume daily life activities that feel right to you.

Focus on your breathing and posture as ways to minimize stress on your body. Start to slowly add in movement such as walking, daily tasks and exercise with intention and without symptoms. Symptoms could include any pain, leakage, feelings of falling out or pelvic heaviness, or coning or bulging at the linea alba (vertical line and connective tissue in middle of your rectus ab muscles). You will want to consider modifying or avoiding activities that bring these symptoms on until you've had time to heal and/or decide to seek out professional help for treatment.

Return to sex when you feel ready. Make it intentional, include good communication and lots of lubricant, and only proceed if pain-free. If it is painful, you can follow many of the tips in the sexual health chapter of this book to reintroduce gentle, positive touch. If you encountered any scar tissue (from tearing, episiotomy, or cesarean surgery during birth), there are ways to improve your sensation and mobility of tissues in this area once things have healed.

MENOPAUSE

Menopause is a natural phase of life that begins after you stop menstruating. The average age of menopause is 51 years old. Menopause is typically defined as a year or longer without menstruation or ovulation. Menopause could happen sooner for a variety of reasons such as a hysterectomy or hormone regimes. It's also possible to go into menopause but then return to a fertile state.

Perimenopause occurs before menopause when the ovaries start to make less estrogen. You usually start noticing a tapering off or less regular periods during this time. Postmenopause are the years after menopause when estrogen production has decreased.

> Any big hormonal shift within our body such as menopause, opens a door within us to choose a path of health or decline. If a person chooses healthy habits at this point in life, it creates a larger effect that ripples deeper into the body than any other time in life. (Erica Macrum, LMT)

Many people may feel differently about this transition. Some people may be relieved not to have their period, or they may feel grief at the end of their childbearing ability, or fear that it means they are no longer attractive, or joy at entering a new phase of self-growth and wisdom. All these feelings are normal, and if you want to talk to someone, there are mental health providers who specialize in this time of life.

As we age and arrive at menopause, there is a natural decline in our bone and muscle mass. You can fight this progression by staying on top of fitness by including regular cardio, strength training, and balance exercises into your life. Find ways that you enjoy moving, make it social, and make it convenient. If you need some tips, work with a local physical therapist or fitness professional. Find ways to fit in moderate aerobic activities most days of the week or vigorous activities a few days a week. Small walks and other forms of movement add up. Also, consider adding resistance training to your mix at least three days a week if possible.

During menopause you may also notice some changes in vaginal dryness, hot flashes, mood swings, weight gain, among other symptoms. It is a natural series of events, but if any of these symptoms are bothering you, consider asking for help. A pelvic physical therapist may be a good choice in searching for education about your pelvic floor changes and setting up a fitness routine.

Some tips for a conservative approach to hot flashes and nights sweats from the North American Menopause Society include:

- Exercising
- Avoiding or decreasing caffeine and alcohol
- Stress reduction
- Maintaining a healthy diet
- Getting quality sleep
- Dressing in layers
- Laughing
- Deep breathing

Because hormones are changing during menopause, consider asking your primary provider if doing a hormone panel may be appropriate for you. It's worth having a conversation about better understanding of your hormones and usefulness of supplementation naturally or medicinally. Hormone replacement therapy has benefits and risks. Make sure you feel thoroughly informed and supported during this decision-making process. Talking with your primary provider or alternative healing practitioners (acupuncturists, naturopaths, and herbalists) about treatment options for menopause-related symptoms would be a great idea.

Take time to slow down and regroup on your health and wellness choices during this time and give yourself some compassion and grace during this transition. Menopause symptoms tend to be easier in cultures where elders are respected and more difficult in cultures that worship youth and devalue age and wisdom.

Consider taking the Menopause Rating Scale (link in the Resources Appendix) to further calculate your current symptoms and share the results with any professionals you may be working with to help get answers and treatment.

LIFETIME CHANGES REVIEW

Our bodies change as we age. Most of it is a normal, natural progression like menstruation and menopause. However, not all the symptoms associated with these changes are pleasant (vaginal dryness, hot flashes). If some of the potential changes are concerning to you or are interfering with your function and quality of life, there may be steps to prevent or treat these changes. Knowing what is normal within these changes and what is not can help you determine if you need to make changes or modifications in your life and/or reach out to a professional for help and guidance.

RECAP

1. Periods are the process of your uterus shedding its lining on a monthly cycle if an ovum has not been fertilized. Normal periods aren't painful.
2. Pregnancy and childbirth change your body. Understanding the changes your body may experience and bringing awareness to your breath and pelvic floor muscles (among other things) can help improve your experience.
3. Menopause is a natural hormonal change, but it can affect your pelvic floor region, strength, bone mass, and more. Being proactive and reaching out for help if needed is a great idea.

CHAPTER 6:

SURGERIES, POP, AND DRA

BEFORE AND AFTER PELVIC AND ABDOMINAL SURGERIES

At some point in your life, you or someone you know may need to undergo a pelvic or abdominal surgery. In most cases, working with a pelvic floor physical therapist prior to and after surgery could help improve your outcomes. There is strong evidence to support this for certain surgeries and little to no evidence for other surgeries, but I'll explain why it might be worth your consideration either way. The pre- and post-op pelvic physical therapy has been shown to be helpful for surgeries including endometriosis excision, hysterectomy, prolapse repairs, cesarean births, gender affirmation surgeries, hernia or diastasis recti repairs, and basically any surgeries involving the pelvic and/or abdominal region.

In pre-op pelvic floor PT, you may learn about how the surgery could affect your pelvic and abdominal tissues and muscles. There may be suggestions to improve your bladder, bowel, and pelvic function to the highest possible level before having surgery. You can improve your awareness of your pelvic floor, your breathing habits and posture, which may help you in your post-op recovery.

In post-op pelvic floor physical therapy, you may work on scar tissue sensitization (decreasing hypersensitivity and/or getting the feeling back if you are experiencing numbness) and mobility of the scar (for better movement) once the scars have healed. You will most likely work on gentle exposure to touch and movement so that you are able to return to all desired functional and leisure activities. You will probably learn how to reconnect with your pelvic floor muscles (strengthen, relax, coordination) and breathing. You will work on returning to all your daily life goals with less pain and better mobility so that you can have an improved quality of life.

PELVIC ORGAN PROLAPSE (POP)

When the pelvic floor (involving both the muscles and connective tissues) weakens, there's a possibility that the pelvic organs (bladder, uterus, and rectum) can descend in the vagina or in the rectum. When these organs descend to the point of creating a bulge in the vagina or rectum, this is called pelvic organ prolapse. Even after a hysterectomy, some people still get a prolapse from the bladder, rectum, or the vagina itself descending in the vagina.

A prolapse is common, but it's not normal. Depending on the degree of this descent and your symptoms, you may want to consider conservative treatment with a pelvic floor physical therapist. Another useful tool before exploring surgical options would be the use of a pessary. A pessary is a device inserted into the vagina to reduce the bulge of the prolapse and help to create support in keeping your pelvic organs up and in. Usually, your first trial with a pessary would be using one that you can take in and out yourself, and you might only use it during times you would be symptomatic (during exercise for example) and take it out in times you don't feel the prolapse. If symptoms are recognized early, pelvic floor physical therapy and pessaries can both be excellent conservative options.

Pictured below are variations of pelvic organ prolapse in a person with a vagina. Prolapses within the rectum are also possible.

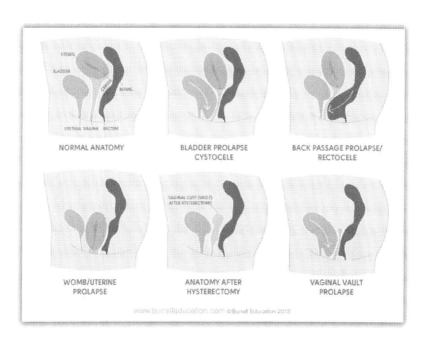

Illustration courtesy of Burrell Education. Used with permission.

Prolapse may feel like

- There's pelvic heaviness or fullness.
- A tampon is falling out.
- There's a bowling ball pressing down.
- Something is coming out of your vagina or rectum/anus.
- You may actually see something like a bubble or bulge sticking out past the vaginal or anal opening.

Pelvic organ prolapse can happen for a variety of reasons: weight gain, pregnancy, childbirth, genetics, nutrition, chronic constipation, chronic coughing, increased pressure. or difficulty controlling pressure on the pelvic organs or quality of connective tissues and gravity.

The more you can do to strengthen and prevent excessive pressure on the pelvic floor, the better chance you have at potentially preventing or treating prolapse.

To prevent prolapse from worsening or to attempt to prevent it from occurring:

- Modify or avoid exercises and movements that cause any of the above symptoms.
- Avoid breath holding and straining regularly.
- Try to maintain regular bowel movements and avoid constipation.
- Learn how to perform your pelvic floor exercises correctly (both contraction and relaxation).
- Perform pelvic floor contractions as a brace before coughing, sneezing, or exerting effort.
- Consider what role nutrition plays with the quality of your connective tissue.
- Get help from a professional such as a pelvic floor physical therapist trained in treating prolapse.

DIASTASIS RECTI ABDOMINUS (DRA)

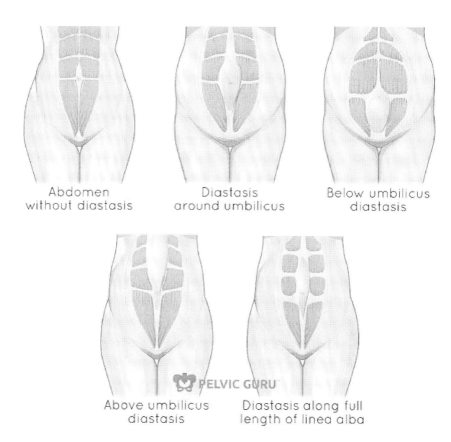

Variations of Diastasis Recti

Abdomen without diastasis

Diastasis around umbilicus

Below umbilicus diastasis

Above umbilicus diastasis

Diastasis along full length of linea alba

Permission to use copyright images from Pelvic Guru, LLC

Diastasis recti abdominus (DRA) is an excessive separation width (greater than two finger widths) or separation depth (sink in without feeling much tension), of left and right rectus abdominis muscles (six-pack muscles) at the linea alba (the connective tissue between the two). The linea alba connective tissue runs from the sternum down toward the pubic bone. The abdominal muscles aren't supposed to be touching. There is a small natural separation between the rectus abdominus muscles. This area is meant to separate as a pregnant belly expands, so it is considered normal during the end of pregnancy.

However, there are concerns for DRA when you are noticing pain or discomfort that interfere with your function and quality of life. If you are seeing doming, bulging, or coning along the linea alba while exercising or moving your body *and* you are experiencing pain or difficulty, you may want to reach out for help.

There are some things that might make this gap worse than what is natural, and it's important to pay attention to your own specific symptoms and experiences with

- Exercises and movements based on your form, load, or duration
  - There are not any specific exercises you *should* or *should not* do just because you have DRA. Everyone will experience different needs for modifications. Please reach out for professional feedback if you are unsure.
- Some postures depending on your form, load, or duration
  - It's great to move in all different ways, but notice if certain postures cause you symptoms.
- Frequent breath holding especially with load
  - Does this increase any symptoms for you?

If you are concerned about DRA due to functional or aesthetic reasons, consider treatment with a physical therapist or fitness professional who specializes in this. An individual approach will be most helpful in figuring out what exercises and modifications will be beneficial to you.

RECAP

1. Pelvic physical therapy can be helpful before and after pelvic and abdominal surgeries.

2. Pelvic organ prolapse can happen when the pelvic organs begin to descend in the vagina or rectum. The good news is there are ways to potentially prevent and to treat prolapse symptoms.

3. Diastasis recti abdominus can happen as your body changes and expands or with pressure system issues, among other causes. You can potentially minimize, prevent, or treat DRA if there are symptoms associated with it that are causing you problems.

FINAL WORDS

The more we know about our bodies, the better we are able to prevent some pelvic dysfunctions from happening or at least lessen the symptoms and impact on our quality of life. If we know what is healthy versus what may be of concern, we are more likely to feel empowered to reach out and ask for help sooner rather than waiting or feeling uncomfortable and unsure.

We all deserve to be happy in our bodies and as healthy as possible. There are many complicated things affecting your health: the society you live in, your access to quality health care, good food and clean water, environmental pollution, and more. My goal is that with resources like this, we can at least change our knowledge about our bodies. The more we talk about, share, and support one another through all health concerns including your pelvic health, bladder, bowel, and sexual health and lifetime changes, the more we improve our well-being and the health of others.

Soak in the knowledge. Ask questions. Keep learning. Share with others. Talk about it openly. Talk about it positively without shame.

Xo Jen

www.facebook.com/jentorborg

@jentorborg_ on Instagram

www.jentorborg.com

DID YOU ENJOY THIS BOOK?

It would be really awesome if you would leave a review on Amazon so others can find out if this book would be helpful to them.

I truly appreciate you taking the time to do that.

ACKNOWLEDGEMENTS

Using my platform to empower others would not be possible if it weren't for:

- The contributions of those who paved the way: Tracy Sher, Susie Gronski, Heather Edwards, Jaime Goldman, Julie Wiebe, Amy Stein, Jessica Drummond, Shelly Prosko, Antony Lo, Sara Reardon, and many more.
- The guidance of Jasper Moon.
- The mentorship of Meagan Peeters-Gebler.
- The UW-La Crosse PT program and especially my partner in all things pelvic, Kelly Diehl.
- All of my wonderful clients I've had the pleasure of working with.
- All the support of my family and friends, especially my awesome husband, Alex!

Many of the following links use cisnormative language in their titles and content. I myself am learning how to correct my own content so that I use trans-competent and inclusionary framework. I hope to eventually change all my content and encourage others in pelvic health to do so that we are not needlessly and harmfully gendering the body.

Find a Pelvic Health Professional near you (more than just PTs) — Global Directory

- Pelvic Guru - https://pelvicguru.com/directory/

Find a pelvic PT near you (USA)

- American Physical Therapy Association Section on Women's Health PT locator - http://pt.womenshealthapta.org/
- Herman & Wallace | Pelvic Rehabilitation Institute - https://pelvicrehab.com/
- Virtual Pelvic Wellness sessions available at The Vagina Whisperer - https://thevagwhisperer.com

Links to those providing quotes and support

Introduction

- Melissa Pintor Carnagey, LBSW, founder of Sex Positive Families - http://sexpositivefamilies.com/
- Intersex Society of North America - http://www.isna.org/

Chapter 1: Anatomy and Physiology 101

- Great Wall of Vagina - http://www.greatwallofvagina.co.uk/home
- The Labia Project - http://www.labiaproject.com/
- Jasper Moon, CPM, LMT - https://www.growingseason.care/
- Pelvic Guru - https://pelvicguru.com/
- Heather Edwards, PT of Vino and Vulvas™ - http://www.vinoandvulvas.com/crotch-coloring-book
- Julie Wiebe, PT - www.juliewiebept.com
- Online courses - http://www.juliewiebept.com/products/online-courses/
- The diaphragm pelvic floor piston demo https://www.youtube.com/watch?v=mLFfZfm7O7c
- The diaphragm and the internal pressure system https://www.youtube.com/watch?v=cW9mwfy-6-I

Chapter 3: Optimizing Bowel Health

- The Flower Empowered - https://theflowerempowered.com/bristol-stool-scale/
- Kate Scarlata, RDN - https://www.katescarlata.com/ https://www.katescarlata.com/fodmaps-101
- Squatty Potty - https://www.squattypotty.com/
- Pelvic Guru - https://pelvicguru.com/
- Dr. Susie Gronski, DPT, PRPC, WCS, WHC - http://drsusieg.com http://drsusieg.com/blog/4-ways-to-a-healthier-gut

Chapter 4: Sexual Health

- Melissa Pintor Carnagey, LBSW, founder of Sex Positive Families - http://sexpositivefamilies.com/
- Sex Positive Families Resources - http://sexpositivefamilies.com/resources/
- Health Line: LGBTQIA Safe Sex Guide - https://www.healthline.com/health/lgbtqia-safe-sex-guide#why-we-need-it
- Human Rights Campaign Foundation: Safer Sex for Trans Bodies - http://assets2.hrc.org/files/assets/resources/Trans_Safer_Sex_Guide_FINAL.pdf
- Planned Parenthood: Sex and Relationships - https://www.plannedparenthood.org/learn/sex-and-relationships
- Epiphora "Your Genitals Deserve Better: the Case Against Toxic Sex Toys" - https://heyepiphora.com/2017/08/your-genitals-deserve-better-the-case-against-toxic-sex-toys
- Ohnut - https://ohnut.co/

Chapter 5: Changes through the Lifetime

- Melissa Pintor Carnagey, LBSW, founder of Sex Positive Families - http://sexpositivefamilies.com/
- Nicole Jardim, The Period Girl - https://nicolejardim.com/ https://nicolejardim.com/four-phases-of-your-menstrual-cycle/
- Period Repair Manual by Lara Briden, ND - https://www.larabriden.com/period-repair-manual/

- Dr. Sallie Sarrel, PT, ATC, DPT - https://salliesarrel.com/ http://endometriosis.org/news/opinion/five-things-that-pelvic-health-physical-therapy-can-do-to-improve-your-endometriosis-related-pain/
- Dr. Jessica Drummond, DCN, CNS, PT - https://integrativewomenshealthinstitute.com/ https://integrativewomenshealthinstitute.com/pcos-pelvicpain-nutrition/
- Link for The Pelvic Pain Natural Relief Method™ https://integrativewomenshealthinstitute.com/opt/4-challenges-to-relieve-pelvic-pain/
- Put a Cup in It:Menstrual cup comparison chart - https://putacupinit.com/chart/
- Menstrual cup quiz - https://putacupinit.com/quiz/
- Party in my Pants - https://partypantspads.com/
- THINX - https://www.shethinx.com/
- Your Best Pregnancy Ever - https://www.amazon.com/dp/1720824487
- Your Best Body after Baby - https://www.amazon.com/dp/1725926776
- Jasper Moon, CPM, LMT - https://www.growingseason.care/
- Erica Macrum, LMT - www.wellbeingupnorth.com
- Menopause rating scale - http://www.menopause-rating-scale.info/evaluation.htm

Chapter 6: Surgeries, POP, and DRA

- Burrell Education - www.burrelleducation.com

- Pelvic Guru - https://pelvicguru.com/

ABOUT THE AUTHOR

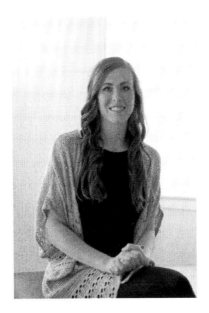

Photo credit: Kelsey Lindsey

My name is Jen Torborg. I'm a licensed physical therapist with a passion for pelvic floor physical therapy. My goal is to empower you on your journey to understanding your body and mind better during all phases of your life and while dealing with pelvic, bladder, bowel, and sexual dysfunction. I was drawn to pelvic health physical therapy because there are sensitive issues in which I feel I am meant to serve. I want to help make a positive impact with this population and increase the public's knowledge about pelvic physical therapy.

This book is my third book in my pelvic floor physical therapy series. My first book, *Your Best Pregnancy Ever*, was published in June 2018, and my second book, *Your Best Body after Baby*, was published in August 2018. Both are available on Amazon through Kindle, paperback, and Audible.

I received my doctorate of physical therapy (DPT) from University of Wisconsin-La Crosse. I have my Certificate of Achievement in Pelvic Health Physical Therapy (CAPP-Pelvic) and Certificate of Achievement in Pregnancy/Postpartum Physical Therapy (CAPP-OB) from the American Physical Therapy Association (APTA) Section on Women's Health (SoWH).

I strive to provide a positive, comfortable environment to treat clients in Ashland, WI at St. Luke's Chequamegon Clinic. I also work with clients virtually through pelvic wellness sessions at The Vagina Whisperer. I look forward to educating my clients about their body and how they can take control of their health.

Outside of my career, I have a love for the woods and the water. I live in the Chequamegon Bay region of Lake Superior. Home to me is being surrounded by trees and trails with the love of my life, Alex, our daughter, Rowan, and our two dogs, George and Lucy. I enjoy being in nature, which gives me a sense of calm and restores me. I love minimizing and tidying. And I'm inspired by beautiful sunrise and sunset.

Printed in Great Britain
by Amazon

42757657R00061